Colour-Blind Superpowers

Living with colour blindness, embracing the challenges, and discovering the superpowers within the disability.

Content

Introduction

Ok, so if, like me, you were diagnosed with being colour-blind at an early age, then the following would resonate with you. If I had a pound for every time fellow students asked me, **"What colour is this pen?"** or **"Why have you coloured that tree in purple?"**, I probably wouldn't have needed to write this book!!

From the early colour-blind tests where you had to find the number hidden within the coloured dots (the Ishihara test), to trying out new ways to beat the colour-blind obstacles in life, I have experienced it all. But I feel that we colour deficiency folk have some incredibly exceptional skills that others don't have and this needs to be explored and celebrated.

Living with colour blindness can be a bit like navigating a world designed for someone else. Whether you are colour blind yourself or a parent of a child who is, you may have faced your fair share of challenges. But what if I told you that being colour-blind isn't just a limitation? It can also be a superpower—a unique way of experiencing the world that brings unexpected strengths and advantages.

This book is about embracing the reality of colour blindness, not just as something to work around, but as a distinctive way of seeing that has its own set of benefits. Sure, there are challenges, like mixing up clothes, or the awkward moment when someone points out the "green" you confidently called "red." But there are also surprising upsides that can make you see this condition in a new light.

We will explore everything from everyday life and practical tips, to how colour blindness can shape careers, hobbies, and even relationships. And yes, we will also delve into the science that explains why some people see colours differently—and why that's not always a bad thing.

This book aims to help you see the beauty in a world that is not defined by the full colour spectrum. Let look into what it really means to live with colour blindness, with all its ups, downs, and hidden superpowers.

Chapter 1: Understanding Colour Blindness

Colour blindness is not just about seeing the world in shades of grey. In fact, the majority of colour-blind people can still see colour, but they perceive it differently from those with typical vision. So, what is colour blindness, really?

What is Colour Blindness?

Colour blindness, or colour vision deficiency, affects the way some people perceive certain colours. Most commonly, it makes it difficult to distinguish between reds and greens, or blues and yellows. Total colour blindness, where someone sees the world only in black, white, and shades of grey, is quite rare.

There are three main types of colour blindness:

1. **Red-Green Deficient (Deuteranomaly):** The most common form, where reds and greens appear similar. For example, a bright red apple might look more brownish green.

2. **Blue-Yellow Deficient (Tritanopia):** Less common, this affects the ability to differentiate between blues and yellows. A blue sky might

appear almost white, or a bright yellow daffodil could look almost grey.

3. **Total Colour Blindness (Monochromacy or Achromatopsia)**: Extremely rare, where all colours are perceived as varying shades of grey.

The Science Behind It

Colour blindness is usually inherited, passed down through genes. It often runs in families, especially affecting males more frequently than females. This is because the genes responsible for colour vision are located on the X chromosome, and since men have only one X chromosome (as opposed to women who have two), they are more likely to experience colour vision issues.

Our eyes contain photoreceptors called cones, which are sensitive to different wavelengths of light corresponding to red, green, or blue. In people with typical colour vision, these cones work together to help perceive a full range of colours. In colour blind individuals, one or more types of cones don't function as they should, leading to the altered perception of colours.

Breaking Down the Myths

There are a few common misconceptions about colour blindness that can lead to misunderstandings:

- **Myth 1: Colour-blind people see the world in black and white.** While complete colour blindness exists, it is rare. Most people with colour blindness can still see colours, just not in the same way others do.

- **Myth 2: Colour blindness is just an inconvenience.** The reality is more complex. It can impact daily life, education, career choices, and even social interactions.

- **Myth 3: Colour blindness only affects men.** Although more common in men, women can be colourblind too, especially if both of their X chromosomes carry the gene.

Personal Stories: Discovering you are colour-blind

Many people don't realise they're colourblind until later in childhood or even adulthood. It is often in school that a child is first identified as colour-blind, perhaps struggling to tell apart colour-coded charts or mixing up the green and red crayons.

For parents, it can be a surprising discovery, often raising concerns about how their child will cope with tasks others take for granted.

But for every story of frustration, there is one of resilience. Children quickly learn to adapt, using context to help them identify colours or relying on friends and family to confirm tricky hues. Some even find creative ways to work around their condition, turning what might seem like a limitation into a unique way of approaching life.

What It Means to be Colour-Blind

Being colour-blind is not just about seeing colours differently; it's about living differently. You learn to navigate the world in ways that aren't dependent on colour. You pick up cues from shapes, textures, and patterns more acutely than most. You might not see the world the way others do, but that does not mean you see less—it just means you see differently.

Chapter 2: The Chemistry of Colour Blindness

Colour blindness isn't just a visual quirk; science shows it may come with hidden strengths. This chapter dives into the fascinating research, evolutionary theories, and recent studies that explore how colourblind brains process information differently, leading to potential advantages.

Research on Pattern Recognition

Studies have shown that colourblind individuals often excel in pattern recognition. Without relying on colour cues, the brain adapts by becoming more attuned to shapes, contrasts, and textures. This heightened sensitivity to patterns can be an advantage in tasks that involve detecting irregularities or visual anomalies. For example, in fields like quality control, data analysis, or even wildlife spotting, being able to focus on the underlying structure of objects rather than colour gives colourblind individuals a unique edge.

One famous hypothesis, the "camouflage-breaking hypothesis," suggests that people with colour blindness are better at seeing through camouflage. Since camouflage often relies on blending colours into the environment, the absence of distraction from colour makes it easier to detect shapes and outlines, allowing colourblind individuals to see through visual deception. This theory has been explored in fields like military research, where detecting hidden or camouflaged objects can be critical.

Evolutionary Theories

From an evolutionary perspective, colour blindness may have conferred certain advantages to our ancestors. In ancient environments where survival depended on spotting predators or finding food, being less distracted by colours could have made it easier to detect movement or changes in texture. Some scientists propose that individuals with colour blindness may have had an advantage in hunting or detecting hidden dangers in their surroundings, allowing them to see things that others couldn't.

Additionally, in early human societies, where foraging for food was vital, colourblind individuals might have been better at spotting fruit or edible plants based on their shape or position rather than colour, particularly in dense forests or grasslands. This subtle advantage could have contributed to their survival, helping them gather resources more effectively in visually complex environments.

What the Latest Studies Are Revealing

Recent research has uncovered new insights into how the brains of colourblind individuals process visual information differently. While the lack of certain colour receptors (cones) in the eyes leads to a different perception of colour, the brain often compensates by enhancing other visual abilities. For instance, studies show that colourblind individuals might process spatial information more efficiently, allowing them to make sense of their surroundings using cues like depth, contrast, and luminance.

Neuroscientific research also reveals that the brain's adaptability, known as "neuroplasticity," plays a role in helping colourblind people develop alternative methods for interpreting visual information. This ability to adapt can enhance overall cognitive flexibility, making it easier to adjust to new environments and visual challenges.

In addition, some studies suggest that people with colour blindness may be better at distinguishing between subtle shades of grey or identifying shapes under low-light conditions. This advantage could be linked to how their brains prioritise information that isn't dependent on colour, making them more adept at seeing differences in texture, brightness, or motion.

Chapter 3: The Daily Struggles and Little Wins

Living with colour blindness is a bit like playing a game where the rules change without warning. Everyday tasks that most people take for granted can become little puzzles to solve. Whether it's choosing the right clothes, reading a map, or distinguishing traffic lights, there are plenty of moments where colour blindness can catch you off guard. But for every struggle, there are also little victories—creative ways to adapt, humorous moments that bring a smile, and unexpected benefits that make you see the world a bit differently.

Colour Confusion in Daily Life

Let's face it—colour is everywhere, and it's often used as the primary way to differentiate things. For someone with colour blindness, this reliance on colour can make certain tasks frustrating. Here are some of the common everyday struggles:

- **Choosing Clothes**: Matching clothes can feel like navigating a minefield. Is that shirt green or brown? Does it match these trousers, or am I about to create a clashing disaster? Many people with colour blindness develop systems, like organising clothes by texture or grouping outfits that definitely go together, to avoid mismatches. Some even use helpful apps that identify colours or get a trusted friend or family member to double-check their choices.

- **Cooking and Food**: Colour plays a role in cooking more than you might think. From checking if a piece of meat is properly cooked to determining if a banana is ripe, colour blindness can make things tricky in the kitchen. However, learning alternative ways to assess food readiness, like feeling the texture of meat or squeezing fruits for ripeness, can be effective. Plus, recipes that rely more on time and temperature rather than visual cues can be a lifesaver.

- **Traffic Lights and Signs**: Navigating traffic can be stressful, especially when it comes to distinguishing red, yellow, and green lights. While most people rely on colour, someone with colour blindness might have to remember the order of the lights (top to bottom) or rely on shapes and brightness to interpret the signals. This can feel daunting at first, but with time and practice, it becomes second nature.

- **Maps and Charts**: Colour-coded maps, graphs, and diagrams are common in school and work environments. For someone with colour blindness, deciphering these can be challenging. Strategies like using high-contrast markers, adjusting the settings on digital maps, or asking for assistance can help make these visual tools more accessible.

Finding the Humour in It

There are plenty of moments when colour blindness leads to amusing situations. For example, there's the classic tale of mismatched socks, when what seemed like two red socks turn out to be one grey and one green. Or the time you confidently described a "red" car, only to learn it was orange.

Humour can be a powerful tool for dealing with colour blindness. Laughing at the mix-ups can make the condition feel less like a limitation and more like an interesting quirk. It can also help others around you feel more comfortable asking questions and learning about colour blindness. Sharing these moments with friends and family not only lightens the mood but can also create a sense of connection and understanding.

Turning Frustration into Adaptation

Every struggle brings an opportunity to adapt. Over time, people with colour blindness develop techniques to work around their challenges. Here are some examples of practical adaptations:

- **Relying on Context**: When colour isn't clear, context can often provide clues. If you can't tell whether a fruit is ripe based on colour, consider its texture, smell, or even the time of year. When dealing with clothes, stick to basics and neutral tones that are easy to match, or label items with tags that indicate the colour.

- **Using Technology to Your Advantage**: Technology has come a long way in helping those with colour blindness. There are apps that can identify colours, adjust screen settings for better contrast, and even simulate how different forms of colour blindness might perceive an image. Tools like these can be especially helpful in situations where colour is important, such as graphic design or digital presentations.

- **Asking for Help Without Shame**: There is no harm in seeking a second opinion. Friends, family members, or colleagues are usually more than happy to lend a hand. In fact, asking for help can sometimes open up interesting conversations about colour blindness, spreading awareness and understanding.

Small Victories and Everyday Wins

Living with colour blindness may come with its set of challenges, but there are also many small victories worth celebrating. These little wins often involve finding creative solutions, turning potential frustrations into accomplishments, or even just embracing the condition's lighter side.

- **Finding Your Style**: Despite the difficulties in matching clothes, many people with colour blindness develop a distinct sense of style. By sticking to simpler colour schemes or creating a wardrobe of pre-coordinated outfits, fashion can become less of a daily struggle and more of an expression of personality.

- **Learning to Cook by Feel, Not Just Sight**: Some people with colour blindness become excellent cooks by relying on other senses, such as smell, taste, and touch, rather than visual cues. Techniques like timing, texture, and temperature can become second nature, turning cooking into an enjoyable experience rather than a chore.

- **Navigating the World Differently**: You might not see the world the way others do, but you learn to interpret it in ways that others don't. Whether it's memorising the order of traffic lights, identifying fruits by their shape, or using contrast to read charts, these adaptations become unique strengths over time.

- **Building Empathy and Understanding**: Living with a visible challenge like colour blindness can foster a deeper sense of empathy towards others facing different kinds of struggles. It helps build patience, understanding, and resilience—not just in yourself, but in the people around you as well.

Embracing a Different View

The reality of living with colour blindness is that it can make you more resourceful and adaptable. What initially seems like a struggle often turns into an opportunity for growth. You learn to see the world in your own way, which gives you a unique perspective that others may not have.

While there are undoubtedly moments of frustration, there are also countless opportunities to discover creative solutions and share experiences that connect you to others. Those little wins—the ones that make you smile or help you overcome an obstacle—are worth recognising. They're proof that while you might see the world differently, you're also equipped to navigate it in your own special way.

Chapter 3: The Colour-blind Superpowers

Colour blindness might not be the first thing that comes to mind when you think of superpowers. However, living with it often leads to unique strengths and advantages that many people without the condition may never develop. The challenges of navigating a world designed for full-colour vision can foster skills that become second nature, and in some cases, colour blindness can offer a different way of perceiving the world that proves surprisingly advantageous.

This chapter explores how colour blindness can be a kind of superpower—an alternative way of seeing that comes with its own set of benefits.

Enhanced Pattern Recognition

When you can't rely on colour, you naturally start to notice other visual cues. Shapes, patterns, textures, and contrasts become more significant. This heightened awareness can be a huge advantage, especially in tasks that require identifying subtle differences or spotting irregularities.

For example, some people with colour blindness have been found to detect camouflage more effectively than those with typical vision because they're less distracted by the colours. Instead, they focus on shapes and patterns that stand out. In fields like the military, this skill can be extremely useful, allowing individuals to see beyond the colour and notice things others might miss.

In everyday life, enhanced pattern recognition can come in handy in various ways, such as recognising faces, reading maps with intricate lines, or noticing when something is slightly out of place.

Thinking Outside the Colour Box

Colour blindness often forces you to develop creative solutions to everyday problems, leading to an innovative mindset. Since relying on colour isn't an option, you learn to use other indicators, such as position, context, or labelling, to make sense of the world. This ability to adapt can foster a type of problem-solving that's resourceful and flexible, which is a valuable skill in any situation.

For example, instead of memorising colours in a game, you might focus on the shapes or placement of the pieces. This can give you an edge in certain strategy-based activities where recognising patterns or changes in shape is more important than identifying colours.

The need to work around colour blindness can nurture a habit of approaching challenges from different angles, a skill that translates well into areas like engineering, design, or even everyday problem-solving.

Resilience and Adaptability

Living with colour blindness teaches resilience. When faced with obstacles like interpreting colour-coded information, navigating social situations, or working in environments where colour plays a major role, you develop coping strategies. Over time, this builds adaptability and a mindset that embraces change.

You become skilled at finding ways to make things work, even if it means taking a different route or using a less conventional approach. This resilience extends beyond dealing with colour blindness; it can help you manage other life challenges with greater ease, as you're already accustomed to navigating a world that wasn't designed with your specific needs in mind.

A Unique View of Art and Design

People with colour blindness often perceive art and design in ways that others don't. Since they see colours differently, their approach to aesthetics can be unconventional and intriguing. Many colourblind artists have created remarkable works by focusing on contrast, composition, and form rather than traditional colour schemes.

This unique perspective can also influence design choices in other fields, such as interior decorating, fashion, or graphic design. By relying more on textures, patterns, and shapes, people with colour blindness can create visually striking designs that stand out precisely because they don't conform to typical colour expectations. In a world where colour is often overemphasised, this approach can feel refreshing and innovative.

Avoiding Visual Bias

Seeing the world differently means that certain visual biases don't affect you in the same way. For instance, while others may be influenced by bright, flashy colours in marketing or packaging, you're less likely to be swayed by these factors and can focus more on the practical or functional aspects of a product.

This ability to look past colour-driven influences can lead to more objective decision-making.

This trait is especially useful in fields like forensics or data analysis, where being able to focus on details that aren't colour-dependent can help avoid mistakes. In some cases, people with colour blindness may spot things that others overlook precisely because they're not distracted by the colours.

Building a Stronger Memory

Without the luxury of using colour as a memory aid, many people with colour blindness develop stronger memories for other details. This might involve remembering the order of things, the shape of an object, or the location of items based on non-colour cues. For example, you may learn to recognise traffic lights not by colour, but by their position on the signal, or identify clothes by their fabric rather than their shade.

Developing these memory skills can be a hidden advantage, as it sharpens your ability to recall information without relying on visual aids. This can be especially beneficial in tasks that require remembering sequences or spatial arrangements, making you more adept at problem-solving or multitasking.

Enhanced Empathy and Understanding

Living with colour blindness can make you more aware of the limitations others face, fostering empathy. You're more likely to understand what it's like to navigate a world that wasn't designed with you in mind, which can extend to a greater appreciation of the struggles others encounter. This awareness often leads to stronger social connections, as people sense that you're someone who truly understands what it means to face daily challenges.

Learning to See the World Differently

The experience of colour blindness teaches you that there is more than one way to perceive the world. Just because you don't see colours the same way doesn't mean your perception is any less valid—it's simply different. This mindset can make you more open to diverse perspectives in other areas of life as well, fostering a broader understanding of the world around you.

You learn to appreciate the subtleties that others might miss, whether it's the play of light on a surface, the shape of a shadow, or the way certain textures catch your eye. In this sense, colour blindness can enrich your experience of the world, offering a form of visual diversity that is truly unique.

The Science Behind the Superpower

Research suggests that people with colour blindness may have evolved specific advantages that helped our ancestors survive. Some studies propose that reduced sensitivity to certain colours could have made it easier to spot predators or prey camouflaged in dense foliage. This idea, known as the "camouflage-breaking hypothesis," suggests that the ability to detect subtle shifts in texture or movement might have provided an evolutionary edge. Marine Biological Lab History

While we no longer need to hunt for survival, this heightened sensitivity to patterns and shapes remains a potential strength. Modern tasks like data analysis, quality control, or anything involving attention to detail may benefit from this inherited trait.

Chapter 5: The Upside of Being Colourblind

Living with colour blindness may present challenges, but it also brings surprising benefits that many might not expect. There is a unique strength in seeing the world differently, and this chapter explores some of the ways in which colour blindness can offer distinct advantages, from building stronger problem-solving skills to fostering a unique sense of creativity.

Enhanced Focus on Detail

When you can't rely on colour to identify objects, you naturally start to notice other details more acutely. Texture, shape, size, and contrast all take on greater importance. For someone with colour blindness, this heightened focus on detail often becomes second nature.

For example, in fields that involve pattern recognition, such as architecture, quality control, or even certain forms of art, noticing fine details can be a valuable skill. By paying closer attention to elements like structure, lines, and shadows, individuals with colour blindness can develop a keen eye for aspects that others might overlook.

Creative Advantages in Art and Design

Artistic expression doesn't have to be limited by colour vision. In fact, some colour-blind artists have turned what others see as a limitation into a source of inspiration. By focusing on contrast, composition, and form, these artists often create works that are distinctive and thought-provoking.

Colour blindness can encourage artists to experiment with unconventional techniques or develop a unique style that sets their work apart. By using textures, bold contrasts, and alternative materials, they can evoke emotions and tell stories in ways that go beyond traditional colour palettes. This approach not only pushes creative boundaries but also makes art more accessible to a diverse audience.

A Different Approach to Problem-Solving

Colour blindness encourages alternative ways of thinking. When you can't depend on colour as a primary identifier, you learn to approach problems from different angles. This adaptability is an asset in many situations, from everyday tasks to complex problem-solving scenarios.

For instance, in situations where colour-based cues are less effective, you might focus on spatial relationships, patterns, or contextual information. This approach can lead to creative solutions that are both practical and innovative, making it easier to tackle challenges that involve more than just visual perception.

Reduced Influence of Visual Biases

In a world full of bright advertisements, flashy packaging, and colourful marketing, people with colour blindness often experience less influence from visual distractions. When colour is less of a factor, you're more likely to make decisions based on practical features, such as quality, functionality, or price, rather than being swayed by the allure of a bright label.

This objectivity can extend to other areas as well, such as evaluating data, judging appearances, or even choosing products. The ability to focus on what truly matters without being misled by surface-level aesthetics can be a hidden strength in many decision-making processes.

Sharpened Memory Skills

Without being able to use colour as a reference, people with colour blindness often develop stronger memory skills to compensate. For example, you might learn to remember where objects are based on their shape, size, or location rather than their colour. Similarly, traffic lights can be identified by position (top, middle, bottom) rather than by relying on colour recognition.

These memory techniques can become valuable in various areas of life, helping you recall sequences, memorise complex patterns, or remember specific details without the need for visual aids. This adaptability not only helps in managing everyday tasks but also strengthens cognitive skills that benefit other areas of life.

Unique Perspective in Scientific and Analytical Fields

In scientific research or analytical fields, a different way of seeing can lead to innovative discoveries. Colour blindness can provide an advantage in areas where pattern detection, shape recognition, or spotting subtle changes are more important than colour distinctions.

For instance, some studies have shown that people with colour blindness may be better at noticing irregularities in textures or shapes, which can be useful in fields such as forensics, biology, or quality assurance. This ability to see past the distractions of colour can open doors to unique insights that contribute to solving complex problems.

Empathy and Advocacy for Accessibility

Living with colour blindness often means experiencing firsthand what it's like to navigate a world that isn't fully accessible. This awareness can foster a deeper sense of empathy for others who face different challenges. It also empowers individuals to advocate for greater inclusivity and accessibility in areas like design, education, and public spaces.

Colour blind people can bring valuable perspectives to discussions about accessibility, ensuring that environments, materials, and experiences are more inclusive for everyone. Whether it's suggesting changes to classroom materials, improving the usability of websites, or designing products that accommodate various visual needs, their insights help make the world more accessible.

A New Appreciation for the World's Subtleties

When you see colours differently, you notice subtler aspects of your surroundings. Light, shadows, textures, and contrasts all stand out in ways that others might not appreciate. This alternative perspective can add a layer of richness to your experience of the world.

For some, colour blindness can even change the way they engage with nature or explore their environment. You might notice the intricacies of a tree's bark or the varying intensities of light on a cloudy day in ways that others don't. These observations, though not reliant on colour, still offer a beautiful and unique view of the world.

Chapter 6: Career Paths and Opportunities

Choosing a career path can be influenced by many factors, and colour blindness is one of them. While some jobs require normal colour vision, there are plenty of fields where colour blindness is not a barrier—and can even be an asset. This chapter explores the ways in which colour blindness can affect career choices, highlights strategies for navigating the job market, and shares success stories of individuals who have excelled in various fields despite or because of their unique vision.

Navigating Career Limitations

Some careers have specific requirements for colour vision due to safety or technical demands. Fields like aviation, the military, and certain medical professions may have restrictions. For example, pilots need to distinguish between different lights on the runway, and electricians must accurately identify coloured wires. These restrictions can feel discouraging, but it's important to remember that there are still many paths open to those with colour blindness.

In cases where colour vision is tested as part of the job requirements, it's essential to check the specific standards for that field. Some jobs may allow for a degree of colour vision deficiency, while others may have alternatives, such as roles that don't involve tasks requiring accurate colour perception.

Success Stories from Unexpected Fields

Despite the limitations in certain professions, there are many examples of colourblind individuals who have excelled in careers you wouldn't expect. Here are some inspiring stories:

- **Art and Design**: While it might seem counterintuitive, there are colourblind artists and designers who have made significant contributions. They often focus on contrast, shape, and form, using their unique perspective to create innovative works. Colour blindness can even become part of their artistic identity, with some artists embracing their condition as a distinguishing feature of their style.

- **Engineering and Technology**: Many roles in engineering and tech don't require perfect colour vision.

In fact, some colourblind individuals excel in areas like software development, mechanical engineering, and data analysis, where recognising patterns and solving problems are more important than identifying colours.

- **Entrepreneurship and Leadership**: Many colourblind individuals have found success in business, leading companies or starting their own ventures. In these fields, the ability to delegate tasks that involve colour-sensitive work can mitigate the challenges of colour blindness, allowing them to focus on strategic decision-making and leadership.

Using Colour Blindness as an Advantage

In some fields, colour blindness can actually be a benefit. For instance, people with colour blindness may have a better ability to detect camouflaged objects because they aren't distracted by the colours and can focus on textures and shapes. This skill can be valuable in roles that involve detecting anomalies, such as quality control, forensic analysis, or even certain aspects of wildlife conservation.

Additionally, colour blindness can foster a mindset that values alternative approaches to problem-solving. Being accustomed to working around a condition like colour blindness can encourage creativity and out-of-the-box thinking—traits that are highly valued in fields like marketing, project management, and product design.

Finding Suitable Career Paths

Here are some career areas where colour blindness is less of an issue, or where the condition can be adapted for:

- **Writing, Editing, and Publishing**: These fields don't require normal colour vision and are ideal for those with strong language skills. Content creation, journalism, and book publishing are all great options.

- **IT and Computer Science**: Careers in coding, cybersecurity, data analysis, and software development rely on skills other than colour vision. In fact, people with colour blindness often bring a unique perspective to data interpretation.

- **Health and Fitness**: While certain medical careers may pose challenges, roles such as personal trainers, physiotherapists, and nutritionists are often accessible. These jobs focus on fitness, wellness, and health education, which don't depend heavily on colour discrimination.

- **Business and Management**: Entrepreneurship, project management, and leadership roles often involve strategic thinking, negotiation, and decision-making. Delegating colour-dependent tasks to others can help overcome any potential limitations.

- **Trades and Craftsmanship**: Many hands-on roles like carpentry, plumbing, and mechanical work can be suitable. While some aspects may involve colour, they often rely on tools, techniques, or safety measures that don't depend on colour vision.

Overcoming Workplace Challenges

For those working in fields where colour can still be a factor, there are strategies to help mitigate the effects of colour blindness:

- **Technology and Tools**: Using software that adjusts colour contrast, apps that identify colours, or wearing special corrective lenses can assist with tasks requiring colour perception.

- **Asking for Reasonable Adjustments**: Don't hesitate to ask for workplace accommodations, such as colourblind-friendly materials, adjusted lighting, or high-contrast displays.

- **Delegating Colour-Based Tasks**: In team settings, assign tasks involving colour matching or identification to colleagues with normal colour vision, while focusing on other responsibilities that utilise your strengths.

Turning Limitations into Opportunities

Living with colour blindness doesn't mean limiting your career options. It means finding opportunities where you can thrive by using your unique skills and perspectives. By focusing on your strengths, learning to work around challenges, and embracing the advantages of seeing the world differently, you can build a fulfilling and successful career.

Chapter 7: Coping Strategies and Practical Solutions

Being colour blindness involves navigating challenges in daily life, but there are plenty of practical strategies and tools available to make things easier. From adjusting your environment to using technology, this chapter offers actionable advice for handling the impact of colour blindness effectively.

Everyday Adaptations

Finding ways to work around colour-related tasks can make daily life smoother. Here are some practical adaptations:

- **Organising Clothing**: Simplify your wardrobe by sticking to neutral tones or buying clothes that coordinate easily. Label clothes with tags indicating their colours or sort them by outfit combinations. Apps that identify colours can help, but relying on known combinations can simplify the process.

- **Cooking Without Colour**: In the kitchen, colour can indicate food readiness, like whether meat is fully cooked. Use tools like meat thermometers instead of relying on colour, and remember to choose recipes that emphasise timing rather than visual cues.

- **Navigating Traffic Lights and Signs**: This may seem an obvious point if you are a regular driver, as our brain is hard-wired to remember sequences that may have a life-or-death outcome. We all know the sequence of traffic lights (red on top, amber in the middle and green on bottom), but under certain low-light conditions these could blur and cloud vision and judgement. So, being familiar with an area during the daytime will help you with the situation in different conditions.

In some cases, wearing colour-corrective lenses can enhance contrast, making lights more distinguishable. But always check with an Optician before driving with corrective lenses.

Leveraging Technology

Advances in technology have made living with colour blindness more manageable. Here are some ways to use tech to your advantage:

- **Apps That Identify Colours**: Mobile apps can detect colours using your phone's camera, providing instant feedback. This can be especially helpful in unfamiliar situations, like shopping for clothes or identifying paint colours.

- **Colourblind-Friendly Software Settings**: Many devices now offer accessibility settings that increase contrast, adjust screen colours, or convert images to high-contrast versions. These features can make digital tasks easier.

- **Colour-Corrective Glasses and Filters**: Special lenses are available that help enhance colour perception for some types of colour blindness. Although they may not work for everyone, they can improve the visibility of certain colours and are worth experimenting with.

Modifying Your Environment

Adjusting your surroundings can make colour blindness less of a barrier:

- **Use High-Contrast Labels and Markers**: Label items with high-contrast stickers or large print to identify important details. For example, use bold black text on a white background to label file folders or kitchen containers.

- **Arrange Items by Shape or Texture**: Instead of relying on colour, organise things by shape, size, or texture. This can be helpful in both personal spaces and work environments, such as distinguishing tools or office supplies.

- **Make Use of Lighting**: Proper lighting can enhance contrast and help differentiate between similar colours. For instance, using daylight bulbs in the kitchen or workspace can improve visibility.

Dealing with Social Situations

Explaining your colour blindness to others can help them understand and offer support:

- **Let People Know When Colour Is an Issue**: If you're working on a project that involves colour-coded materials, communicate your needs clearly. People are usually understanding and willing to make adjustments, such as using patterns or symbols in place of colours.

- **Use Humour to Break the Ice**: Lightening the mood with a humorous remark about colour confusion can make social interactions smoother. It helps others feel comfortable and fosters a supportive atmosphere.

Embracing Tools and Support Systems

Don't hesitate to seek support when needed:

- **Find Online Communities for Colourblind People**: Sharing experiences and tips with others who understand your situation can be encouraging.

- Online forums and social media groups often offer valuable insights on coping strategies and new technology.

- **Seek Reasonable Accommodations in the Workplace**: If your job involves tasks where colour is critical, discuss accommodations with your employer. Simple changes, like using alternative labelling or adjusting screen settings, can make a big difference.

Chapter 8: Psychological and Social Implications

Living with colour blindness goes beyond practical challenges; it also affects emotional well-being and social interactions. Understanding the psychological and social aspects of colour blindness can help build resilience, foster a positive self-image, and encourage openness in social situations.

Emotional Impact: Frustration, Embarrassment, and Anxiety

Colour blindness can sometimes lead to feelings of frustration or embarrassment, especially when you struggle with tasks others find simple. Whether it's mixing up colours in social settings, or dealing with misunderstandings, these moments can cause anxiety. It's important to recognise that these experiences don't diminish your worth or abilities—they're simply part of navigating a world designed for colour vision.

Coping with Feelings of Frustration

Here are some strategies to help manage emotions related to colour blindness:

- **Practice Self-Compassion**: Accept that colour blindness is just one aspect of who you are. It doesn't define your capabilities or value.

- **Use Humour to Diffuse Tension**: Laughing at mix-ups can turn potentially awkward situations into light-hearted ones, making it easier for others to understand.

- **Reframe Challenges as Learning Opportunities**: When you encounter difficulties, see them as chances to develop problem-solving skills and build resilience.

Building Confidence: Embracing Colour Blindness as Part of Your Identity

Accepting colour blindness as a unique aspect of your identity can empower you to approach life with confidence. Embrace it not as a flaw, but as a different way of experiencing the world. Here are ways to instil a positive mindset:

- **Focus on Strengths and Achievements**: Recognise the areas where you excel, and don't let colour blindness overshadow your successes.

- **Share Your Experiences Openly**: Talking about colour blindness with friends, family, or colleagues can demystify the condition, reducing stigma and building understanding.

Navigating Social Situations

Colour blindness can be tricky in social contexts, where assumptions about colour perception are common. Here's how to handle these moments:

- **Be Open About Your Condition**: Mentioning colour blindness casually can help set expectations. It's okay to ask for help or suggest alternative ways of doing things.

- **Use It as a Conversation Starter**: Sharing stories about your experiences can spark interesting discussions, raising awareness and creating opportunities for connection. I do this on a regular basis in my work environment or when I am having to public speak. Remember colour blindness is a disability which shouldn't define you. You need to define it and make it work in your favour.

The Role of Support Networks

Connecting with others who understand the challenges of colour blindness can be comforting. Whether it's online communities or local support groups, having people to share tips and experiences with can make a difference.

Turning Colour Blindness into a Source of Empathy

Experiencing the limitations of colour blindness can foster empathy for others facing different challenges. This awareness can help you develop deeper social connections and advocate for inclusivity.

Chapter 9: Colour Blindness and Creativity

Colour blindness can inspire creativity in unexpected ways, challenging traditional approaches to art, design, and problem-solving. Far from being a limitation, it can unlock new forms of expression that rely on contrast, composition, and texture. In this chapter, we'll explore how colourblind individuals channel their unique vision into creative pursuits, reshaping how they engage with visual media.

Rethinking Colour in Art

For artists with colour blindness, creating visual art often involves a different focus—on contrast, light, and form. Since traditional colour palettes are less reliable, these artists turn to bold lines, striking shapes, and play with textures to evoke emotion or tell a story. Colour becomes secondary, while other visual elements take centre stage.

Some colourblind artists have embraced their condition by developing distinct styles that challenge the conventions of colour-based art. By using alternative materials, focusing on grayscale or monochromatic schemes, or experimenting with strong contrasts, they have turned colour blindness into a defining feature of their creative identity.

Innovative Approaches in Design

Colourblind designers are known for their ability to think beyond conventional colour theory. They may rely on patterns, shapes, and layout to communicate ideas effectively, creating designs that are more accessible and impactful. In industries like graphic design, architecture, and product design, the focus often shifts from creating visually appealing colour combinations to ensuring clarity, functionality, and accessibility.

For instance, in web and interface design, colourblind designers are more likely to prioritise usability over aesthetic concerns, making them naturally inclined toward inclusive design principles. Their attention to detail in areas like font choice, spacing, and layout can result in products that are intuitive and easy to use for everyone, regardless of their vision.

Expanding Visual Thinking

Living with colour blindness encourages a broader view of visual thinking. Since the condition forces individuals to rely on cues other than colour, they develop a heightened awareness of depth, texture, and balance.

This can lead to innovative approaches in disciplines beyond art and design, such as photography, film, and even fashion. Colourblind photographers, for instance, may focus on contrasts of light and shadow to create striking, atmospheric images.

In fields like interior design or fashion, where colour is often key, colourblind creatives find ways to adapt. They might rely on advice from others, but ultimately their designs reflect a deep understanding of composition, texture, and harmony.

Breaking the Rules of Traditional Colour Theory

One of the advantages of colour blindness is that it encourages breaking the "rules" of traditional colour theory. Without being constrained by conventional perceptions of complementary or analogous colours, colourblind creatives are often more willing to experiment with unusual combinations or monochromatic schemes that challenge expectations. This freedom leads to fresh and original work that doesn't fit within standard norms.

Success Stories from Colourblind Creatives

There are many examples of successful creatives who have turned their colour blindness into a defining feature of their work. Some renowned artists, designers, and photographers have embraced their condition, creating iconic work by focusing on elements other than colour.

These individuals demonstrate that creativity transcends limitations, proving that vision is about much more than just colour. I personally used to paint and sell my art in my younger days, and it always amazed me that more people didn't question the colours I was using in my art. This was always a confidence booster to me. But sometimes made me question if I was still colour blind or if I had somehow been cured (which is of course not possible!).

Chapter 10: Technological Advances and Looking to the Future

The future looks bright for those living with colour blindness, thanks to ongoing technological advancements and scientific research. From innovative tools to potential treatments, new developments are changing the way people with colour blindness navigate the world.

Innovative Tools and Corrective Technologies

One of the most significant advancements in recent years has been the development of colour-corrective glasses and lenses, such as EnChroma. These glasses use special filters to enhance colour perception for people with certain types of colour blindness, allowing them to see colours more vividly. While these lenses don't cure colour blindness, they can provide a much richer visual experience for users in specific environments, such as outdoor settings or with digital screens.

Beyond lenses, there are also apps that help colourblind individuals identify and differentiate colours.

Mobile apps like Color Blind Pal or See Colors use a phone's camera to analyse and label colours in real-time, offering instant assistance in everyday situations like shopping, cooking, or matching clothes.

Genetic Research and Future Treatments

Scientists are making exciting progress in the field of genetic research, exploring the possibility of correcting colour blindness at the genetic level. Gene therapy is one of the most promising areas, particularly for individuals with inherited colour blindness. This experimental treatment involves modifying the genes responsible for the condition, potentially restoring normal colour vision.

While these treatments are still in the early stages of research and not widely available, the potential to "cure" colour blindness in the future is becoming more of a reality. Clinical trials in animals have shown promising results, and human trials are expected to follow as the technology advances.

Accessibility in Design and Education

The growing awareness of colour blindness has led to significant improvements in accessibility, especially in design, technology, and education.

More companies are now recognising the importance of designing products and interfaces that are accessible to people with colour vision deficiencies. Websites, software, and digital platforms are increasingly incorporating colourblind-friendly features, such as high-contrast modes, patterns instead of colours, and clearer labelling.

In education, there is also a push toward more inclusive learning materials. Teachers and curriculum developers are becoming more mindful of how they use colour in visual aids and resources, ensuring that students with colour blindness are not left out or confused by colour-coded charts, graphs, or maps.

The Future of Inclusivity and Innovation

As technology continues to evolve, the world is becoming more accessible for people with colour blindness. There is a growing movement toward universal design, which benefits everyone, regardless of their vision abilities. From user-friendly interfaces to public spaces designed with inclusivity in mind, the future looks promising for more accommodating and thoughtful designs across industries.

At the same time, ongoing scientific research holds the potential for breakthroughs that could fundamentally change how colour blindness is understood and treated. Whether through new tools, corrective treatments, or groundbreaking therapies, the future is full of possibility for individuals with colour blindness.

Chapter 11: Conclusion and Final Thoughts

As we come to the end of this journey, it's clear that living with colour blindness is about more than just navigating a world designed for full-colour vision. It's about adapting, finding strengths where others see limitations, and embracing a unique way of experiencing life. From enhanced pattern recognition to innovative problem-solving, colour blindness can be a superpower, offering skills that many people never develop.

Throughout this book, we've explored the challenges and triumphs of living with colour blindness, from everyday tasks to larger career and lifestyle implications. More importantly, we've uncovered the ways in which colour blindness can be embraced as a strength—a way of seeing the world differently, with distinct advantages in creativity, adaptability, and perspective.

As science and technology continue to evolve, the future for people with colour blindness looks even brighter. From advanced corrective lenses and accessibility tools to potential genetic therapies, the world is becoming more inclusive and accommodating. But perhaps the most significant takeaway is that colour blindness doesn't need to be "fixed"—it's simply another way of perceiving the world.

Whether you're colour blind yourself or supporting someone who is, remember that this condition isn't a barrier to living fully and creatively. It's a reminder that there's more than one way to experience beauty, solve problems, and contribute to the world. Embrace your unique view of life, and let it become a source of pride and strength.

Resources for Support and Information

- **Colour Blind Awareness**: (www.colourblindawareness.org) – A UK-based organisation offering support, educational materials, and advocacy for colourblind individuals.

- **Colour Blindness in Children**: (www.colourblindawareness.org/children) – A resource for parents to better understand and support children with colour blindness.

- **The Colour Blindness Foundation**: (www.colourblindnessfoundation.org) – Information and global awareness efforts focused on colour vision deficiencies.

Recommended Tools and Apps

- **EnChroma Glasses**: Glasses designed to enhance colour perception for people with certain types of colour blindness (www.enchroma.com).

- **Color Blind Pal**: A mobile app that helps identify colours by using your phone's camera.

- **Chromatic Vision Simulator**: This app allows users to see the world as someone with different types of colour blindness.

Frequently Asked Questions

1. **Can colour blindness be cured?**
   - While there is no cure currently, corrective glasses and ongoing genetic research offer promising options for improving colour perception in the future.
   -

2. **Is colour blindness common?**
   - Yes, around 1 in 12 men and 1 in 200 women worldwide are affected by colour blindness.

3. **How does colour blindness affect children in school?**
   - Colour-coded materials can pose challenges, but teachers can use alternative methods like patterns, symbols, or labels to make learning more accessible.

I hope you have enjoyed and got what you need out of the tips and advice from this book. I also hope you can see that being colour deficient doesn't make you different or less worthy than those with (normal) sight. To be honest is anyone ever normal? That is a question for a later topic!

www.ingramcontent.com/pod-product-compliance
Lightning Source LLC
Chambersburg PA
CBHW071217260726
48653CB00041B/888